# 2econd Chance

## A Journey to Rediscover Inner Strength

NICOLE L. BEVERLY

Cover Photo: Ryan Mitchell

Cover Design: Branford Brown

Copyright © 2017 Nicole L. Beverly

All rights reserved.

ISBN: 978-0-578-60119-9

# DEDICATION

To Dad and Mom, thank you for your love, guidance, and friendship. You are my best friends and cheerleaders. My will to make a difference is strong, because I've witnessed the difference both of you have made in the lives of others.

To my close friends, thank you for teaching me to speak my truth and to pursue my dreams no matter how long it takes for them to come true.

Lastly, to those who have a story of strength and survival, share your experience to help others. Knowledge is freedom and it is meant to be shared, not hoarded.

# CONTENTS

Introduction                                i

1   The Blueprint                          Pg 1

2   False Evidence                         Pg 5

3   Denial. Acceptance. Denial.            Pg 7

4   Knocked Down, but not Out              Pg 11

5   Get Off the Couch                      Pg 13

6   Back to Basics                         Pg 18

7   Purge and Cleanse                      Pg 24

8   The Brilliance of Simplicity           Pg 28

9   The Crossroads                         Pg 32

10  Favorite Health & Wellness Tricks      Pg 34

# INTRODUCTION

I chose to write this book for two reasons. First, writing is a journey in discovery of who we are at different stages in life. Writing provides healing, connection to a higher level of consciousness, and it can be a source of strength as we acknowledge and discard deeply rooted toxic emotions.

The second reason I chose to write this book is because I believe my experiences can be the motivation and strength for others who are struggling to identify what ails them - be it physical, emotional, or mental. As my spirituality has evolved, I know that the steps (and perceived missteps) I take in life are all preordered by God - - it's everything according to His plan. He already knows what I'm going to do, how I will do it, who will be involved, and what the outcome will be. My life experiences shared here are a constant reminder that God is the one in control, not me – as I had so long believed.

Words are extremely powerful and moving for me. Throughout this text there are excerpts from my journal which document my actual moods and random thoughts. To survive my experience I **had** to journal; it was not an option. The excerpts are shown in italicized bold font.

This story is about a several-years long journey to rediscover and reclaim my inner strength through a range of emotional, physical, and spiritual challenges. It's also about cultivating the will to rise above it all, to persevere and to thrive.

My story could've been much different if it were not for the shelter dog I adopted. She gave me a reason to **want** to get better, and she taught me that second chances are sometimes the best gift we could *never* imagine. Because of the profound effect pet adoption has had on my life, 50% of the proceeds from this book will be donated to the Prince George's County Animal Shelter (Maryland) in the form of supplies.

Challenges are part of growth and are not absent from anyone's life. It is my prayer that you or someone you know may find similarities in the challenges I faced, and learn from the steps I took to overcome them. I hope this text will be the catalyst for your courage to heal and move forward in fulfilling God's purpose for your life. **You are a born survivor**.

-Namasté, *The spirit in me honors the spirit in you.*

# 1 THE BLUEPRINT

All my life I've been tiny; petite. As a youngster, the repetitive comments from others were "oh, you're so little, I'll bet you wear a size zero," and on and on. Ironically, I did wear a size zero at one time! How can there be a size nothing? That's just stupid.

Even as an adult people have said to me "you look like you're twelve, I wish I was your size," and blah, blah, blah. I learned early on that some people just don't know what to say, when it's best to say nothing at all.

American society tends to equate a petite stature with fragility, needing to be "taken care of", weakness, lack of authoritative presence, and people feeling like they need to speak for you. I suppose it was these inaccuracies that fueled my formative years and molded my character--my blueprint.

## Strong-Willed

Strong-willed, that's how my parents described me growing up. I recall seeing a book on my Dad's nightstand titled **The Strong Willed Child** by Dr. James Dobson. I was like "Wow, they have to read a book about me?" I wasn't a difficult child in the negative sense. Rather, I always questioned EVERYTHING! I had [and still have] a desire to learn and understand the "why" behind a decision, even from authority figures like my parents. It drove them crazy.

My father often told me "your mouth is going to get you in trouble," but to me, decisions didn't make sense unless they could be backed up with evidence and or logical reasoning. I guess my parents wised up to this, because I can remember only once or twice being told "because I said so". That's not to say I didn't get the occasional butt whipping for being sassy, but the discipline was preceded by a reason.

I dissect, rationalize, and archive every interaction – good and bad. The people who know me best also know they should be prepared with a rebuttal or detailed thought process before engaging in serious debate with me. Hey, someone has to play devil's advocate to keep them sharp!

## Quiet Power

My genetic blueprint is chock full of a blood line that quietly commands respect. Quiet power – that's how a former employer described me. You see, I've always been a reserved person - slow to trigger an over the top reaction. Ok, maybe the one exception was during the teenage years when everything was considered over the top! However, when I have something to say, I speak in a manner that is melodic, well thought out and commands attention. In other words, you'll never see me coming, because there's no need to be loud, bullish or overbearing. I'm secure in my thoughts, beliefs, actions and abilities. I'm also seasoned enough to know when I don't know something, so I'll sit back and learn from others.

As for my personality, it's been described as aloof; intimidating; nonchalant; introverted, yet charming and down to earth. It's an interesting learning opportunity to hear how you are viewed by others. In my case, it's fairly accurate to some degree, but has been refined with age and life experience. Here's how and why.

*Aloof and nonchalant* - These descriptors are attributable to my reserved nature. I'm not easily roused or impressed, so people interpret this as being uninterested. While in fact, I'm selective about who I engage with in conversation, so if we're talking to each other at length, I'm obviously interested in what you have to say. My parents are humble people and that was passed on to me. I don't put on airs for anyone.

*Intimidating* - I'm amazed at how some interpret being reserved and observant as intimidating. I think this is because it's difficult for them to read someone who's not yelling at the top of her lungs, jumping up and down with a "look at me" attitude. I don't need the attention or approval of others to feel validated.

*Introverted, yet charming and down to earth* - Now go figure how in one case someone thinks of me as intimidating, while someone else thinks of me as charming and down to earth. Maybe the difference is the level of self-security between the two people! Life is always about interpretation, isn't it?

I am mostly an introvert, because I find more value in listening to and observing people, rather than being in the spotlight. A dearly departed family friend, Deacon Martin Capehart, frequently said "stand up to be heard, and sit down to be appreciated". I think that perfectly sums up my introverted nature.

On the other hand, I can be an extrovert depending on the situation – public speaking, event hosting, running a business. The bottom line is that there has to be a REASON for me to be in the spotlight.

Charming and down to earth is the core of who I am. My family doesn't subscribe to bad manners or a superiority complex. I was taught to treat everyone with respect, even when respectfully putting them in their place. We are all human and subject to the same imperfections, frailties in judgment, and sins. No one is above God.

My blueprint is what I had to rediscover along this journey in order to reclaim strength and thrive on my own terms.

# 2 FALSE EVIDENCE

Picture it…the year was 2009 *(This is my homage to the character Sophia from The Golden Girls television show. She began every story with "picture it".* This is where my story begins.

Prior to 2009, I had never failed at anything that was really important to me. I had significant academic and work experience, I was financially stable, physically active, a healthy eater, was working fulltime and also managed a part-time business for four years at this point. Then strange things began to happen to me emotionally and physically. Something just wasn't right.

I was 30 years old when weird things started happening to me. I didn't sleep as well as I used to. It seemed like every few months I experienced short durations of extreme fatigue and mild insomnia.

Our health is our most valuable asset. Without it, there's little we can accomplish. When faced with seemingly daunting health concerns, it is human nature to initially regress and seek darkness in which to wallow alone. On the other hand, it is also human nature to fight - - the choice is ours. I chose to fight.

After months of just not feeling like myself, I was encouraged to talk with a counselor about what was going on. At this time, my symptoms were more emotional than anything else, so talking with a mental health professional seemed like a reasonable idea.

## Facing my Fears

I'm a private person when it comes to my thoughts and feelings, so I was reluctant to begin counseling, but I also knew that I needed help, because I didn't have the emotional stamina to heal on my own.

During a series of nine one-hour long sessions, my counselor suggested I get a medical workup to rule out any underlying issues that could've been the reason for my emotional distress and uncontrollable moodiness. I was just sad ALL OF THE TIME and couldn't pinpoint why. I would cry at the drop of a dime for no reason…I mean sobbing to the point my nose wouldn't stop running and my eyes swelled like golf balls! What was going on?

Following the counselor's advice, I visited an endocrinologist to have the lab work done. An endocrinologist is a specialist who treats people who suffer from hormonal imbalances.[1] Emotions are driven by hormones, so it made sense to start here.

---

[1] http://www.hormone.org/contact-a-health-professional/what-is-an-endocrinologist; accessed 24 May 2016.

# 3 DENIAL. ACCEPTANCE. DENIAL.

In June 2009, the results were in. Diagnosis: Hypothyroidism – an underactive thyroid gland. According to www.webmd.com, hypothyroidism means your thyroid is not making enough thyroid hormone.[2] The thyroid gland secretes several hormones throughout the body which support metabolism, body temperature, and growth and development. These are just some of the body's functions that rely on the thyroid.

"Okay, so how do I get rid of these problems" I asked my doctor. He replied "Oh, you'll be on medication for the rest of your life." I was angry; that was not what I wanted to hear. I thought to myself, *"He doesn't know who I am. I'll show him. I'm not taking medication for the rest of my life. I'm going to beat this and I'm going to prove him wrong."*

I swallowed my pride for that moment, scheduled a three month follow-up appointment, and left the office with prescription in hand for my "rest of life" drugs. As I waited at the pharmacy for the prescription to be filled, I was overcome with a flood of emotions and thoughts. How did this happen? Why me? I can't be sick. I'm never sick. How long before I feel better? How long before I get rid of this condition?

My mood changed from sad to defiant and empowered, back to sad. This emotional tug of war went on for weeks.

After the diagnosis, my life and focus changed immensely for the better. I once focused on career and financial prosperity. Now the focus was faith, health, happiness and love - in that order. While career and finances still had a place in my life, they were much farther down the list.

### Hypothyroidism (Hypo) Helped to Organize My Life

For someone who doesn't know me, who doesn't know the complexities of Hypo, and who doesn't have a deep connection to nature, it is difficult to comprehend how I embraced this health challenge, despite how it affected my life.

One might question how acknowledging a seemingly incurable condition that causes muscle and joint pain, extreme fatigue, weight

---

[2] http://www.webmd.com/women/tc/hypothyroidism-topic-overview; accessed 6 August 2015.

fluctuation, and much more, is even a sane approach to dealing with it. Well, my question is this: What was my alternative? At the onset, I could accept Hypo, learn about it, learn how to manage it, and be in control of it. Or, I could allow it to control me.

I don't know about you, but I don't believe in giving up. I fight for the things worth fighting for, and my life and happiness are worth more than any material possessions I've ever owned.

Hypo challenged me head on with brute force. It required me to love myself more than loving possessions and printed green paper with pictures of dead old white men- - that's American money by the way.

Medical challenges force us to place ourselves above worldly cares. Such challenges insert an extended pause in our way of living, affording us an opportunity to reprioritize and reflect on the value of life and all it embodies - gentleness, appreciation and respect for life and nature, kindness toward others, and finding the purpose for our journey.

## Journal Excerpt (undated)

*As I write these words I am in pain. My body hurts and I feel like crying, but I will not be defeated. My purpose is larger than a moment of discomfort. My purpose is to share my experience and educate others on how they can rise above whatever challenge is at their door. Face your challenge, because it is impossible to truly live and be a recluse at the same time. My high school English teacher would call that an oxymoron![3]*

## Journal Excerpt (undated)

*I'm beginning to understand now. Since being diagnosed with hypo, I've become more in touch with and aware of what my body is telling me. I pay more attention to the foods and beverages that my body craves, because they are what my body needs at that specific time. I also pay better attention to what foods my body does not like. For example, excessive caffeine, too many walnuts, red meat, greasy foods, pasta, too much wheat, processed sugar, and the list goes on.*

---

[3] Oxymoron: something (as a concept) that is made up of contradicting or incongruous elements. http://www.merriam-webster.com/dictionary/oxymoron; accessed 28 August 2012.

*Our bodies are drawn to what they need through smell and sight, and that can mean different needs on different days. I don't claim to be an expert on hypo, but I am an expert on myself and how it affects my life. I discovered that I thrive on a high intake of fruits and leafy green vegetables, while keeping animal protein to a minimum.*

What makes your body feel its best? If you don't know, you may have to begin the analysis by keeping a food and beverage journal for at least three weeks. Describe how you feel after eating and drinking each time. The body is extremely intuitive, we just need to learn how to listen to it.

The magnitude of symptoms associated with hypo can make for years of learning how to successfully manage the condition. It took me one year to merely learn and, unwillingly, experience most of the symptoms. I realized that my periods of mild insomnia weren't just because I had a cup of tea a few hours before bed.

There were many nights I never had any caffeine before bed, but still struggled with falling asleep and staying asleep. The insomnia was a symptom of hormonal imbalance, specifically the hormone melatonin. Melatonin is responsible for regulating our body's sleep process. So guess what? Yep, insomnia is a symptom of hypo.

### *Journal Excerpt, 29 August 2012*

*Today is a tough day. I woke up with aches throughout my body. As a result, I feel sluggish, somewhat depressed, and overall disinterested. I recently increased my dosage to help with the achiness, but no relief. This is so frustrating. I feel like I'm rapidly aging. There's so much I want to do, but my body can't keep up.*

### *Journal Excerpt, 30 August 2012*

*After three days on an increased dosage, I've returned to just one pill a day. I feel much less achy today and have a more positive attitude. I had a good 30 minute stretching session today, which helped to loosen my back and hips. Today was a good day.*

### *Journal Excerpt, undated*

*I experienced a breakthrough in determining why my body aches occasionally in every joint. It's all related to my diet. When I'm stressed out or bored, I tend to crave sweets. More often, those sweets are of the processed variety, rather than all natural sweets like fresh fruits, or naturally sweet veggies like raw carrots.*

*I began to notice that within several hours to one day after eating foods made with processed sugar, my body, specifically the joints, would become stiff and achy. This observation led me to conduct my own dietary experiment. I eliminated processed sugar from my diet for one week and immediately noticed that I was free of aches and stiffness, and I sustained energy throughout the day without feeling run down or sluggish by the end of the day. Although it made perfect sense to continue a sugar-free diet, it proved extremely difficult for me to maintain. There's much truth in the adage "some people have to learn the hard way." I relapsed and had a processed sugar binge one weekend; my body paid for it for at least four days afterwards.*

So let's think about what a processed sugar attack is really doing to a body that reacts the way mine did. Let's begin with the obvious yet forgotten fact that the human body is derived of the Earth and in such, it is designed to digest foods that are of the Earth. The human body is not designed to digest fabricated foods. Fabricated foods, also known as processed foods, are those which have been altered from their natural state, resulting in diminished nutritional value, or the complete absence thereof. What sense does it make to eat something that takes away from you being able to perform at your optimal best?

I challenge you to find one person who eats fabricated foods every day for several years and is not suffering from some underlying medical challenge. Good luck with that search.

# 4 KNOCKED DOWN, BUT NOT OUT

In the midst of addressing health concerns, I was now coping with unhappiness and an unfulfilling marriage. I had emotionally divorced myself from the relationship several months earlier. It seemed as though the foundation of stability in all aspects of my life was crumbling around me. In my mind, the marriage issues were another failure because I couldn't fix them, at least not by myself. Although the ex-husband and I made an effort to improve the marriage by going to counseling, a square peg cannot be forced to fit into a circle. We were not on the same page in terms of life goals as partners. It took me a year to come to that realization and finally say enough is enough. I was not satisfied with just existing. I needed to make a difference.

The frustration and disappointment of the revelation that my marriage was going nowhere added to my health issues in the way of mild depression. I had a decision to make. Stay in the marriage and continue to be unhappy, unfulfilled and watch my health decline, or pray for God to speak to my heart and tell me what to do. It was not an easy decision. After all, I'd only been married for a little more than two years at this point. The third year anniversary was approaching, but I was numb. My emotional well was dry.

After months of praying and seeking direction, the need to prioritize is what forced my decision. I had to reclaim my health. Without good health I was no good to anyone, especially myself.

We divorced and I haven't looked back. It was the hardest, yet most necessary decision I've ever made. It was a decision that sparked my new journey toward holistic wellbeing and reinforced my principles of health and happiness before anything else.

Let me be clear, going through a divorce is not without a grieving process. When you commit to joining your life with someone else, losing that promise and dream is like the death of a close loved one. No matter how prepared you think you are for the split, it still hurts and leaves you feeling hollow, perplexed, depressed, unworthy, and lost. While I did not regret leaving the person, I greatly missed married life – coming home to someone, sharing interests, family activities, caring for someone, and so on.

With so many challenges at one time, I'd lost my identity. Towards the end of the marriage, I gave up my small business because I no longer had the passion for it. This was another part of me that died.

My once full schedule outside of work had been replaced with sleeping, eating just enough [junk food] to keep my stomach from growling, and then sleeping some more. I hated how I felt and withdrew from going out and visiting family and friends. It was too hard to pretend to be happy. However, time truly does heal all wounds.

# 5 GET OFF THE COUCH

Grief hit me like a ton of bricks. The last time I felt this bad was when both of my grandfathers passed away. They were the only grandparents I'd known, since one grandmother died before I was born, and the other died when I was too young to remember her.

I was seriously settling into the hermit life. The ultimate couch potato by now, an indentation had begun to form in the sofa!

I lay there day after day, curtains closed shut, and the television on with a TV tray full of junk food and used facial tissues. My house was in disarray, and for those who know me well, that alone was a red flag that things were falling apart. I always took pride in keeping a clean and orderly home, but even that was no longer important to me. I'm embarrassed to admit that I did not even bathe on the weekends - - for what? I wasn't going anywhere. I really just didn't care. *"God help me please"*, I prayed. *"I can't go on like this. When will my heart stop hurting?"*

It was imperative for me to get off of that couch, otherwise things were going to continue to get worse very quickly. Although I never seriously considered suicide, it crossed my mind for a brief moment. Then I thought how such a selfish act would bring so much pain to my family and go against God's commandments. Suicide was not an option.

One day I thought to myself *"What would make me happy right now? I need a REASON to get off the couch. A pet would require that I take care of it. A dog would require exercise, and that would be good for me too."* Right then and there it was settled. I was going to get a dog to force me off the couch.

On March 21, 2012, Skye opened my eyes and I opened my life to her. That March 21st was a beautiful day. The temperature was comfortable and the sun was bright. My mind raced with excitement and nervousness at the same time. I was preparing to pick up the baby I had waited decades to bring home. Her name was Skye and she was the Rottweiler I wanted since childhood.

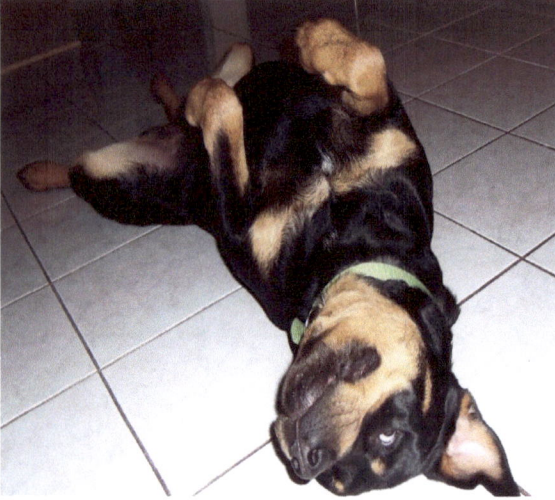

Photo Credit: Nicole L. Beverly

One week prior, I researched the local animal shelter's website and viewed the dogs available for adoption; particularly female Rottweilers.

When I saw Skye's picture and read about her I knew she was the one. Not much was known about Skye, other than she was about three years old, was picked up as a stray, and she had two scars on her back. It was unknown what caused the scars, but the presumption was that she had been abused at some time and the scars were a permanent result. Despite the scars, she had a healthy weight and disposition; her last owner had cared for her. Skye had been at the shelter for about one month.

I had finally decided to live for myself and do what brought **me** happiness. Part of this was getting a dog. Since the age of nine I wanted a dog, but not just any dog. I wanted a Rottweiler. I don't remember what triggered my fierce loyalty and love for the breed, but I do remember it happening at age nine.

I was not allowed to have a dog when I lived with my parents. [Mom and Dad, I get it now. They're a lot of work, money, and commitment, even more so for two working parents with children.]

I can talk about dogs and especially Rottweilers all day long. They are a working breed with origins in the ancient town of Rottweil,

Germany.  Skye, however, is not a working dog…she IS work!  She is my spoiled diva.

Today there are German bred and American bred Rottweilers.  The only real difference is that the German dog is slightly larger than its American cousin.

Rottweilers are highly intelligent and intuitive, which has made them excellent for law enforcement work, guarding, herding and search and rescue.  They were originally bred to guard cattle owners and their herds on the way to and from market, while wearing the owner's money bag around their neck.  No one would dare try to take that money!  They were also known to stand up against bears.

The Rottweiler at home with its family is still protective, but is also calm, gentle with children, a playful clown, extremely sensitive and loving, and wants to be wherever you are at all times.  Because of their size and strength, they must be obedience-trained and socialized early and often with people close to you and with other dogs.

Along with physical exercise, their intelligence requires regular exercise in the way of frequent new activities and opportunities to learn.  Otherwise, a bored Rottweiler becomes a destructive one that is simply trying to release stored up energy and frustration.

I picked up Skye from the shelter on that beautiful March day and brought her home to a second chance with someone who would shower her with love and attention.  I could tell that she'd had a litter of puppies not long before coming to the shelter.  We bonded immediately.  It was amazing how we were so close in just days, and after three weeks, I dared anyone to harm her; they would have to deal with me.  I'm sure she would've conveyed the same if she could speak words.  It was obvious that we needed each other.

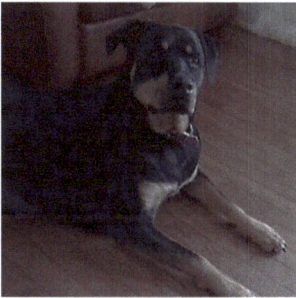

Photo Credit: Nicole L. Beverly

Skye exudes the nobility of the Rottweiler.  She is calm and gentle, yet alert and cautiously curious.  She is loving, clownish, and intuitive. I can "see" her thinking.  She is loyal and protective.  She is even nurturing.  How can a dog be nurturing towards a human you might ask?  Well, one evening I was working on my girlish figure by rocking out some pushups.  At some point I started breathing very heavy - stop laughing at my expense. Skye came over to me and put her nose to my face. She sniffed me, licked my arm and paced from side to side, waiting to see if I was okay. I finally gave in to the muscle fatigue and just laid on the floor. Again, she sniffed me.

I raised my arm and wrapped it around her reassuring "Skye, I'm okay girl, I'm okay." Afterwards, she laid down next to me and remained there until I got my second wind to get up.

Skye's presence in my life has been such a turning point. She is what got me off of the couch. Because of her, I found a reason to believe in love again; to believe that I still have plenty of love to give and am equally well deserving of it.

Observing and interacting with Skye sparked several changes in the way I approach life today. These lessons are basic principles that are applicable to all of us.

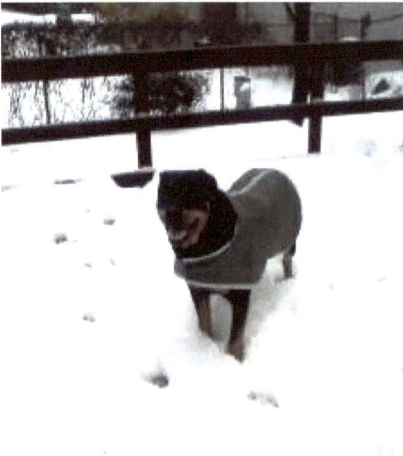

Photo Credit: Nicole L. Beverly

Skye's taught me:
- To speak with gentleness
- To remember how to play and the simple joy it brings
- To cultivate patience (especially when I'm cleaning her ears)
- To explore nature
- To require people to earn my trust and time
- To be loud and clear about what and who I like and don't like; AND I don't need a reason
- To be firm with my rules

- To love unconditionally
- To let the past be the past; deal with an issue then move on
- Love is a powerful healer.
- We CAN be happy with just love, food, shelter and water.
- It's okay if she occasionally eats dead bugs, because I occasionally eat dead chickens! (Of course I'm referring to the chicken we buy and cook!)
- Some people will make assumptions based on your appearance and will never like you, even if they don't know you and you've never done anything to them. Ignorance is wasted thought.

- I have a lot of love to give.
- Health and happiness should always win over money and possessions.

# 6 BACK TO BASICS

Over a four year period I struggled with a chaotic imbalance of emotions, hormones, and prescription dosages for my thyroid. Too many days I felt hopeless, like a failure because I couldn't figure this out! Failure was foreign to me, so I had a really difficult time accepting that the condition was not my fault. Instead, it was a temporary challenge and test of my faith.

While Skye's presence and caring for her brought a great level of joy and purpose to my life, there were days I reluctantly shared my tears, physical pain and overall frustration with my parents about my health challenge. It would've been impossible to hide from them anyway, because they could always tell when something was bothering me.

My day of reckoning had come. I couldn't cry anymore, and I was tired of being sick and tired – literally and figuratively speaking. It was time for real and sustainable healing.

Four years after diagnosis, in May 2013 my mother and I were on one of our usual checking-in phone calls. I don't remember exactly what we talked about, but I'm sure I gave her an update on whatever new ailment was bothering my body. She shared that a friend referred her to a doctor of Naturopathy, and that she had begun to see this doctor with initial good results. At my mother's urging and encouragement, I agreed to schedule an appointment with the doctor.

Later that month I visited the doctor of Naturopathy for an initial one hour diagnostic evaluation. Let me tell you, I was very skeptical of the techniques used, but I also knew that God places people in our lives for a reason, and He gives us everything we need to heal ourselves naturally. So, I was willing to give it a chance. My alternative would've been to continue the same erratic, downward then upward then down again spiral. No thanks, I'd had enough of that.

My first naturopathic visit was very pleasant and full of education. *Did I mention that I love learning? Remember that always needing to know why thing about me...*

Anyway, I was connected to a machine that transmits and receives small electrical pulses via the finger tips. Our body is full of electrical impulses which serve as a conduit of information between the brain and central nervous system – the spinal cord. These impulses carry information throughout the body and back to the brain. Like a well-oiled machine, optimal organ function, nerve function, cellular and muscle function are all dependent upon properly working electrical synapses.

My body and the machine carried on an extensive "conversation" about what was going on with me. This process was a Bio Meridian scan. The rhythm of the conversation was audibly expressed as a series of tones at varying durations. Whenever there was significant imbalance detected in my body, the machine seemed to hum for an extremely long time, collecting a mass of electrically transmitted data. This data was analyzed, compiled and depicted in text and charts on a connected laptop. Bottom line – the process and detailed information provided was out of this world!

I know this all sounds unbelievable, but it's important to note that while connected to the machine, the doctor asked me very specific questions to confirm my symptoms, without me offering any information ahead of time. For example, during one visit, my lower back and thigh muscles were very sore from having worked out just a few days earlier. I did **not** share this with the doctor. Yet during my Bio Meridian scan, the machine communicated data that those areas of my body were experiencing soreness! From that moment I was convinced that this machine was the real deal, and I became a strong advocate of natural medicine. Natural medicine is the world's first medicine; period. It was time for me to get back to basics.

A Bio Meridian scan is just one among several methodologies for the delivery of natural medicine. The website http://biomeridiantesting.com/ defines Bio Meridian testing as *a noninvasive method used to assess the energy meridians (channels) of the body, and it can tell you: the functional status of your meridians and their related organs, systems, or functions, by determining if they are stressed, balanced, or weakened, and by how much.* Some other widely recognized forms of natural medicine are acupuncture, acupressure, aromatherapy, and massage. The list is vast.

How many times have you heard the cliché *knowledge is power*? The more knowledge one has about options for medical care, the more control one has over his or her ability to heal, without introducing counterproductive side effects and toxic chemicals into the process.

Think about it this way. Your body is derived from the Earth; thus, it can quickly recognize and respond to medicinal treatments that are also derived from the Earth. Conversely, when natural treatments are altered or replaced by toxic, man-made chemicals, the body cannot rebound as quickly, nor can it fully eliminate the toxins because they are not recognizable, and toxins are therefore indefinitely stored in body tissue.

If you've never learned or heard someone speak German, would you recognize the language? Of course you wouldn't recognize it. So why would one expect the human body to recognize a language other than its "natural" language – medicine of the Earth? The logic really is this simple. Say what you will about natural medicine, but be certain you are speaking from experience.

My first naturopathic visit revealed that I had a mineral imbalance; not hypothyroidism. A mineral imbalance can present symptoms similar to a thyroid condition. The imbalance was revealed by a hair tissue analysis (HTA).

To begin to rebalance the minerals in my body, the doctor prepared a 90-day treatment plan consisting of herbal supplements [the size of horse pills], a modified diet, and herbal tinctures – herbs that are dissolved in a solution of alcohol.

An HTA test is beneficial in determining the **root cause** of medical problems, because hair follicles retain biochemical information for several months, whereas typical blood tests will only reveal information spanning just hours or a few days old. Why else would certain blood tests require you to fast before lab work can be done? Typical fasting before blood work may last up to 12 hours. How will fasting for several hours produce a blood specimen that will reveal what's been going on in your body for years? It won't. It will only reveal what's been going on for 12 hours!

In my opinion, an HTA is more comprehensive, as it provides a several-months long "history" of the body's condition, which can more accurately pinpoint the root cause of a problem and address it systemically, rather than symptomatically.

I do, however, believe that blood tests have their place in situations such as a sudden onset of infection or in monitoring a pregnancy. These are all situations of short duration; they are acute. However, for chronic situations like severe insomnia, inflammation, cancer, diabetes and lupus, I believe an HTA is more beneficial in order to craft a holistic treatment plan.

I believe Western medicine is consumed with labeling everything that is deemed "not normal", and thereby tries to convince us that we need a prescription to fix this or that. When in fact, it is NOT normal to be chronically ill. However, it IS normal for the body to become imbalanced and sick from time to time, but prolonged imbalance and sickness is NOT normal, nor should it be accepted or masked with toxic medication touted as 'disease management'. *Managing* something implies you want to keep it around. One should manage activities, not diseases. Diseases are to be eradicated; period!

Let's stop medicating our symptoms and instead find solutions so we can get back to living.

Labels give the appearance that it's okay to not feel well, because *we can give you a prescription for that*. I digress…this Western medicine versus Natural medicine is an entire series of books all its own.

## The Turning Point

Over the course of my 90-day treatment plan, I began to reduce the toxins in my body by replacing foods, beverages, and toiletries with their natural and organic version. Instead of just fresh fruit, I bought organic fresh fruit free of pesticides. Instead of fluoride toothpaste, I bought natural fluoride-free toothpaste. Instead of antiperspirant, I bought aluminum-free and fragrance-free natural deodorant. (As a side note, it is natural for the body to perspire; this is how the body keeps cool. So using ANTIperspirant robs the body of its natural function, which creates imbalance.) I also bought body lotions with natural and organic ingredients.

In following the plan and making the change to a mostly natural and organic lifestyle, I slowly began to notice a difference in my energy level, joints and the condition of my hair and skin. My body was beginning to heal and rebalance itself. During the treatment plan, I visited the doctor about once every three weeks for a bio scan to see how things were looking inside my body. My mineral levels had improved and were realigning themselves. We made adjustments to the plan as necessary by removing or adding herbal tinctures.

Needless to say, I have not taken thyroid medication since my first naturopathic visit in May 2013. Today, I continue to rely upon natural medicine for health and wellness, and organic foods for nutrition.

An organic lifestyle can be challenging when it comes to socializing. I have become very picky about eating only organic when it is available, and I don't eat out much anymore because I want to be certain of where my food comes from and how it is handled. Therefore, if I go to an affair at someone's house and I know our lifestyles are different, I will eat before I go. In this manner, I control what's available to eat. There! My secret's out. Now my family and friends know why I never seem to eat much when I visit them. So really, it's not you, it's me!

My lifestyle is my choice. Therefore, it's also my responsibility to ensure it remains intact as much as possible. The goal is to maintain the healthy habits I've developed, not to regress and become imbalanced again. Imbalance leads to an unhappy body and weakened immune system. That would be like putting regular gasoline into a diesel engine – just asking for trouble. No thanks, I don't want that kind of problem.

The other challenge [or annoyance] of a natural and organic lifestyle is that everyone wants to be a critic, or somehow convince me that I'm weird, what I eat *doesn't taste good* or *it's too expensive to eat organic.* First of all, why do they even care what **I choose** to eat? They're not paying for my food or my health bills. Anyway, my response to such criticism is this: I eat for nutrition, not entertainment. Sure, buying organic or growing my own vegetables or fruits may be a little more costly and time consuming, but the alternative to be chronically ill is a lifetime expense of medical bills, toxic medication, and one NEVER gets well. It's much easier and less expensive to stay healthy than it is to *work at becoming healthy.*

I do not believe in forcing my lifestyle upon anyone. Instead, I look for opportunities to educate people on health and wellness. However, that can only be achieved with someone who is willing to receive the kind of knowledge that requires changing and retraining one's thought process. It requires thinking as an individual, rather than as a member of a culture that taunts us with advertisements of mega-sized portions of unhealthy foods and beverages that are always solicited with *having a good time.* I'm not saying deprive yourself of a treat once in a while, but too much of anything is never good for us. Again, one should eat for nutrition, not for entertainment. Healthy eating isn't boring if you know your way around the kitchen.

23

# 7 PURGE AND CLEANSE

Getting back to basics by changing my daily diet and the type of hygiene products I used greatly helped to reverse the physical challenges I experienced. Yet, to be fully "healthy" required looking at my life as a whole. While my body was on the mend, it was just one part of the machine that defines the human species. The other parts are mental and spiritual.

## The Thought of it All

My mental health during this journey was adequate to get me through each phase of healing, but it wasn't as strong as I wanted it to be. In fact, it had some Swiss cheese holes because my spiritual being had been neglected. You see, to me mental and spiritual health are interdependent - one cannot thrive without the other. When I speak of mental health, I'm referring to a holistic spiritual awakening - the cleansing and retraining of thought processes, the purging of toxic relationships, and learning to honor one's personal space and time by setting boundaries with those around us.

While I could speculate for weeks about WHY I did certain things, I needed help from a mental health professional to learn how to break the cycle so I could become a stronger version of myself. Once again, I sought counseling. At this stage in my journey nothing was off the table.

In order to achieve God's will for my life, I had to be at my optimal level of performance. I needed "all hands on deck" and sought wisdom from those with the experience to help me get to the next level.

During this round of counseling, which lasted one year, I discovered why I had such a hard time with the feeling of failure during the hypothyroid diagnosis and during the divorce. As a child, my family experienced nearly losing my brother to drowning. To this day, I remember the look of despair on my Mother's face when she overheard a phone call my Father answered. On the other end of that call was my brother's best friend who said my brother had drowned.

I remember my Mother dropped to her knees in desperation for it not to be true. Thankfully, my brother was revived minutes later when his friend called back with an update. But witnessing my Mother's response, and enduring the events in the hours that followed, was forever etched in my young mind. From that moment on I subconsciously placed a burden on myself that "I had to do everything right. I can't disappoint Mom and Dad, because I don't want to see them hurt." I didn't want them to worry about me the way I saw them worry about my brother.

That one moment in time caused me to be extra critical of everything I did and the choices I made, because I "didn't want to disappoint anyone". So when I encountered a medical issue that was seemingly out of my control, followed by a divorce, I interpreted those experiences as failures because I could not control them. They were disappointments. They were a sign of my weakness – so I thought. What a revelation it was to discover the "why" of how I operated. I had placed so much pressure on myself to be perfect and to not make mistakes. No one can sustain a life free of mistakes.

I also discovered through this counseling that the mental clutter in my head was due to unfinished work. I have a very bad habit of starting lots of things at one time, but never finishing any of them. In this manner, my gift of being a visionary is a blessing and a curse. While I'm skilled at planning and seeing the big picture, I still struggle with the "baby steps" it takes to get to the big picture. I've accepted this about myself and it's taught me to delegate more; personally and professionally. For those things that absolutely must have my attention and mine alone, I have to force my brain to focus on that task until it is done. I'm still a work in progress, but the point is that I'm progressing. I'll never be perfect at this, because that would be like trying to change my DNA. As long as I know how to manage my thought processes in order to focus and accomplish one task at a time, I've already won. Knowing is half the battle, right?

So I identified and learned how to purge deeply rooted behaviors and cleanse my thought processes. The next battle up was that of purging toxic relationships. This was easier for me to do, because I had done it throughout my life. Whenever a personal or professional relationship caused me to act out of character, it was time to bury that relationship. Equally, when it began to feel like I was giving more effort to a relationship than the other person, it was time to say goodbye. That process has not changed for me.

The difference in my relationships now is that I more freely communicate my thoughts and feelings with the other person, rather than assuming they know how I feel and just blowing them off. I also want to hear from them how they interpret my words. If we can clear up a misunderstanding, that's wonderful. Yet, if our individual compasses continue to overlap and constantly redirect instead of intersect, then the relationship's season is over.

Everything in life literally has a season – a time of birth and death – and the cycle repeats itself. I was finally beginning to learn the spiritual aspect of this cycle. God gives us what and who we need at specific times during our journey to mold us into the magnificent person He created us to be. Remember that everything that happens to us is by His divine plan.

The humanity in us sees loss as sorrow. Yet from the existential point of view, we lose nothing; we gain wisdom and strength through experiences.

This was my spiritual awakening. I hadn't failed. In fact, I had overcome and grown smarter, stronger, and more respectful of my spiritual, emotional, and physical health. I was so elated about this new space of personal evolution that I wanted to jump through the roof. I was learning to be at peace with being imperfect.

I no longer dwelled on what should've, could've, or would've been because it was not in God's plan for me. Instead, I focused on what relationships and activities would help me grow and how I could help others. This is the purpose of life as I see it. It's so simple that it's brilliant.

# 8 THE BRILLIANCE OF SIMPLICITY

It is amazing how difficult we can make life just by adding our anticipations of "what ifs" and "if this happens, then I'll do that…" fantasies. Just accept life's challenges as they come without judgment or expectations. When I adopted this behavior, I reduced my stress level and became less reactive to situations, and instead became more relaxed and cleared-headed when making decisions. I became a more evidence based decision maker, rather than an emotionally driven decision maker.

If you're at least 30 years old, you've probably made enough emotionally driven decisions to realize they require a lot of energy. They zap us at our core and drain us mentally and physically. Often they do not produce the results we *anticipated* that they would.

To live simplistically I had to develop and consistently practice a different way of *being present* in my own life. I learned how to be in the moment, rather than always trying to anticipate my next move or that of people around me. This required much introspection and humility to understand that not EVERY moment I experienced was about me. Real life example: one day I was driving home and out of nowhere got a craving for one of my favorite beverages. I wasn't even thirsty, but I stopped at a nearby convenience store to purchase the beverage and noticed a man loitering outside.

He looked frail, his hair was not combed, and his clothes were not clean. Although the weather was not cold, this man was shivering. After I made my purchase, I left the store and popped the trunk of my car to get a blanket out that I kept for emergencies. To me this was an emergency, because at that moment he needed the blanket more than I did. With blanket in hand, I walked up to him and said "Hello. It's a little chilly out here, so I thought you might like to have this. May I buy you something warm to drink?" He said no to the warm drink, but graciously accepted the blanket.

The simplicity of being in that moment is that I made no assumptions about the man, nor did I have any expectations. I simply saw someone in need and offered what I thought would help.

God sent me to that store to help that man at that time. How many people do you think went in and out of that store all day long and never bothered to look twice at the man because of his appearance? How many people do you think offered him anything? I can't remember anything else I did that day, but I remember the man. The fact that he is what I remember is proof that the day was about him and not about me or the activities I had done. It was simply about him.

As I learned to become an evidence based decision maker, I noticed that my anxiety level diminished. I no longer felt the pressure to be perfect in every action. After all, there's no such thing as perfect. We are all perfectly *imperfect*. So let's breathe a sigh of relief together!

Learn to be in the moment and be present in every act and conscious of every decision. Think what you might miss from the present if you're always anticipating the future. Food for thought...a clock can only be ahead of time if **we** push the hands forward. Don't be so anxious to push. Let every minute have its purpose.

I added *more life* to my space by incorporating household plants. Plants not only help to clean the air in our home, they also serve as a constant reminder of life's fragile nature. If we ignore a plant's basic needs it will perish. Yet when we feed and nurture those basic needs, plants flourish and can reach their full potential. I do not have a green thumb, so I selected plants that are easy to manage. I live with a Peace Lilly and Philodendron.

The Philodendron was a learning curve, but after I did some research and adjusted its placement in the house, it has been easy to care for.

The more simplicity I incorporated into daily life, the more at peace I felt. I took stock of my living environment and donated unnecessary stuff like furniture that no longer served a purpose, extra dishes I didn't need, and clothes that hadn't been worn in years. I de-cluttered emotional baggage by shredding paper memories of difficult times; they were now officially buried. Clearing out the visible clutter in my home environment helped to de-clutter my mind. I gradually regained mental sharpness, physical energy, and emotional stability.

I also created a dedicated "my space", which is my yoga room. The room is simple – a yoga mat on the floor, soft light from a small lamp, a wall mounted TV for my yoga and exercise DVDs, minimal wall décor, and a Buddha statue. While yoga is **not** a religion and I do not practice Buddhism, the statue is a reminder of the peaceful nature of yoga and its origins.

## Relax the Mind and the Body Will Follow

I began practicing yoga in 2009 as a way to manage the physical discomfort of the so-called hypothyroid condition I had. Yoga not only helped ease the joint and muscle pain, it also helped me to focus and de-stress. I practiced yoga sporadically until early 2015 when I decided to pursue it more deeply by completing a yoga teacher program. I completed Level I Yoga Teacher training in April 2015. The training taught me the history of yoga, the proper alignment of poses and their health benefits, and to connect the physical aspect of each yoga pose with its spiritual benefit.

Yoga is an ancient practice rooted in India that is more than 6,000 years old. It teaches that the mind, body and spirit are all connected. If one element suffers, the other two become unbalanced. However, when all elements work in harmony, the whole person is in balance. I can attest to this firsthand in that once I finally learned to relax my mind, the tension I'd been holding in my body began to release and permit my muscles and ligaments to relax. Thus, with every practice I was able to stretch deeper into the poses, hold them for longer periods of time, and control the rate and duration at which I inhaled and exhaled.

Yoga can be practiced by people of all ages and abilities. People have been known to practice yoga well into their 90's, and practice sessions can be customized in accordance with a person's health or mobility limitations. It is truly a way of life that teaches us to be in the moment, for one must focus on controlling his or her breath while in each pose. Otherwise, balance will be lost and one can risk injury. Yoga also encompasses various forms of meditation through which one learns to calm and focus the mind.

To this date, whenever I feel overwhelmed or feel tension creeping up in my body, I tell myself to relax and the body will follow. It truly does work, for the mind holds the coding that controls our body. We are God's super computers – correct any glitches in the code and the computer will function as it was intended.

# 9 THE CROSSROADS

My journey since 2009 has enlightened me. While difficult at times, it has been a source of encouragement because I know God has more in store for me. The challenges I encountered over the past several years were not the end of my story; they were the beginning. I emerged stronger and wiser and with real purpose.

At this juncture in life, I am clear about God's plan for me. That doesn't mean I claim to know His plan. It means I accept whatever dreams and passions He places within my heart, for they are part of my purpose and will serve as the continuation of my story.

My dreams are plenty and my passions never-ending. The truth is that both will outlive me, but they will live on through the legacy I build now. Those whose lives I have been blessed to positively impact, along with those who I have yet to meet, will continue to carry the torch I've lit. My purpose is to leave the world better than when I entered it. What good is a life that doesn't serve others?

I never imagined that I would write a book, yet I have because I was destined to live through something so remarkable to me that I felt compelled to share the experience with others. I felt a *passion* to share. I never imagined I would practice or teach yoga, yet I do because it was part of my healing and I know the power it has to help others.

As I stand at the proverbial crossroads, I can't help but feel joyful, inspired, and blessed that God chose me for the story and journey I've shared with you. I made it and you can too! You have the strength deep inside to overcome any obstacle and to achieve greatness in everything you set out to do. We are born for greatness, but it does not happen solely because of our individual efforts.

God did not create us to be alone. With so many people in the world, we exist solely to help and be helped by one another. You are not alone in your current situation. Know that seeking help is a sign of strength, not weakness. It takes a strong person to recognize their limitations in overcoming certain obstacles. To deny oneself the assistance in attacking those obstacles can severely handicap progress towards becoming the magnificent person he or she was born to be.

When you arrive at the crossroads, take the direction in which your shadow appears, because this is the road where God is shining His light upon you for all to behold. This road will have some bumps, ditches, standing water, and many twists and turns. Yet the farther along that you travel, the destination will come into focus and within your grasp. You will emerge taller, stronger and wiser for having had the courage to accept an unknown journey to rediscover inner strength.

Until we meet again…

# 10 FAVORITE HEALTH & WELLNESS TRICKS

Through trial and error over several years, I've perfected some of my favorite health and wellness routines. Some of these might work for you too and are an inexpensive alternative to over the counter products.

***Disclaimer: If you have a skin condition or other medical condition, discuss these tips first with your physician to make sure they are safe for you to use. I have not endorsed any specific brands, so feel free to find a brand that works best for you. Be sure to use organic whenever available.***

Skin and Hair Care
- Core Olive Leaf can be applied topically to minor cuts, acne blemishes, and nail infections. To apply, dip a Q-tip in the Core Olive Leaf then apply to the affected area.

- Raw Organic Shea Butter can be used for healing scars, bruises, and skin health in general.

- Organic Coconut Oil and Organic Olive Oil are good moisturizers for skin, scalp and hair. Use sparingly, as a little goes a long way. If you're allergic to nuts, do not use coconut oil.

- Organic Coconut Oil is a great alternative to deodorant. It absorbs quickly and controls sweat and odor. If you're allergic to nuts, do not use coconut oil.

- Facial Scrub – Make your own facial scrub to use twice per week, year round:
  o Mix 1 teaspoon organic coconut or olive oil, juice of 1 organic lemon, and 1 tablespoon of table sugar. Gently massage the mixture over your face and neck in a circular motion. Rinse with warm water and pat dry. Apply your favorite moisturizer to finish, and remember sunscreen if going out during the day.

- Insanely Soft Arms and Legs Scrub – Use up to twice per week year round. Mix 2 teaspoons organic honey, 2 tablespoons table sugar, and 2 tablespoons of organic coconut or olive oil. The consistency should be thick, but workable. Apply in a gentle circular motion, then rinse with warm water and pat dry.

### Boost Immunity and Treat Colds

1. Take Core Olive Leaf liquid orally to kill infections. Follow dosage instructions on the bottle.

2. For tough colds, swallow 1 teaspoon of Raw Organic Apple Cider Vinegar (with The Mother) three times per day, up to three days per week. The taste will be very strong. If you prefer, mix the vinegar with 6oz of water and drink. Note: Taking the vinegar by itself is more potent and works faster. DO NOT use vinegar if you have ulcers or a severely sore throat.

3. Beginning in September, take liquid Vitamin C with Rose Hip to build immunity for the winter. Follow dosage instructions on the label.

# ABOUT THE AUTHOR

Nicole L. Beverly is a writer, motivational speaker, and entrepreneur. She is a natural health and wellness advocate, having experienced the powerful transformation it made in her life.

Nicole is passionate about sharing her experience with natural healing and holistic living so that others may discover the fullest potential for their lives.

www.ingramcontent.com/pod-product-compliance
Lightning Source LLC
Chambersburg PA
CBHW040345060426
42445CB00029B/4